The Complete Alkaline Diet Cookbook

A comphrensive mix of alkaline recipes for you everyday meals

Isaac Vinson

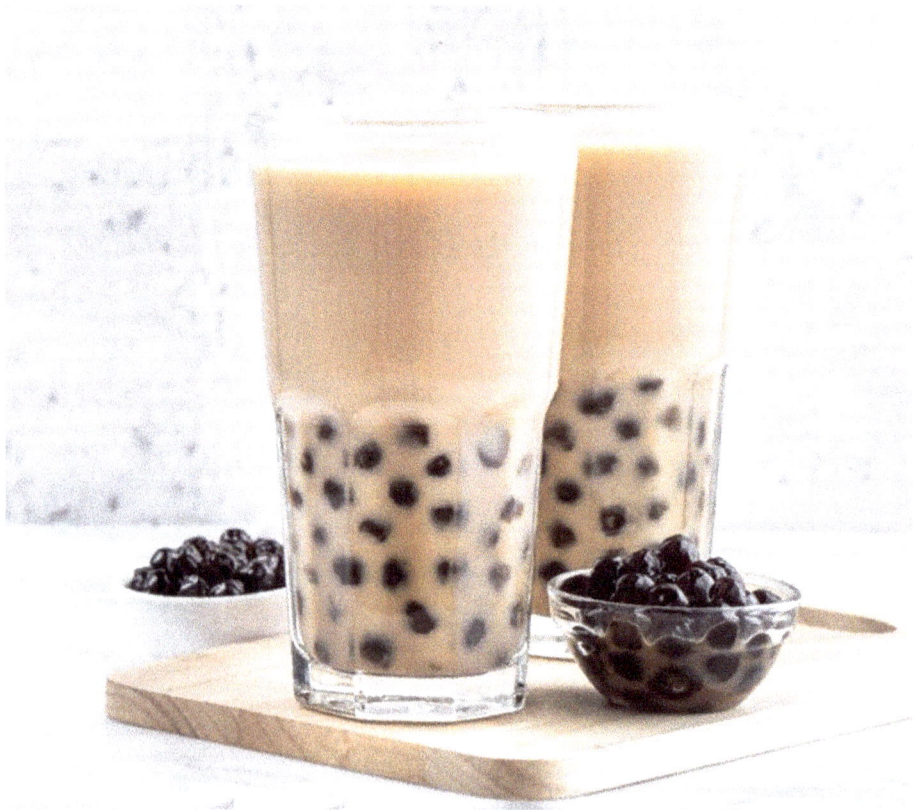

Table of Contents

Energizing Lemon Tea

Preparation Time: 5 minutes

Cooking Time: 15 minutes

Servings: 3

Ingredients :

• Lemongrass, .5 tsp. dried herb

• Lemon thyme, .5 tsp. dried herb

• Lemon verbena, 1 tsp. dried herb

Directions:

Place the dried herbs into a tea strainer, bag, or ball and place it in one cup of water that has boiled. Let this sit 15 minutes. Carefully strain out the tea. You can add agave syrup or date sugar if needed.

Nutrition:

Calories 40

Sugar 6g

Protein 2.2g

Fat 0.3

Respiratory Support Tea

Preparation Time: 5 minutes

Cooking Time: 18 minutes

Servings: 4

Ingredients :

• Rosehip, 2 parts

• Lemon balm, 1 part

• Coltsfoot leaves, 1 part

• Mullein, 1 part

• Osha root, 1 part

• Marshmallow root, 1 part

Directions:

1. Place three cups of water into a pot. Place the Osha root and marshmallow root into the pot. Allow to boil. Let this simmer for ten minutes

2. Now put the remaining Ingredients into the pot and let this steep another eight minutes. Strain.

3. Drink four cups of this tea each day.

4. It's almost that time of year again when everyone is suffering from the dreaded cold. Then that cold turns into a nasty lingering cough. Having these Ingredients on hand will help you be able to get ahead of this year's cold season. When you buy your ingredient, they need to be stored in glass jars. The roots and leaves need to be put into separate jars. You can drink this tea at any time, but it is great for when you need some extra respiratory support.

Nutrition:

Calories 35

Sugar 3.4g

Protein 2.3g

Fat 1.5g

Thyme And Lemon Tea

Preparation Time: 5 minutes

Cooking Time: 10 minutes

Servings: 2

Ingredients :

• Key lime juice, 2 tsp.

• Fresh thyme sprigs, 2

Directions:

Place the thyme into a canning jar. Boil enough water to cover the thyme sprigs. Cover the jar with a lid and leave it alone for ten minutes. Add the key lime juice. Carefully strain into a mug and add some agave nectar if desired.

Nutrition:

Calories 22

Sugar 1.4g

Protein 5.3g

Fat 0.6g

Sore Throat Tea

Preparation Time: 8 minutes

Cooking Time: 15 minutes

Servings: 4

Ingredients :

• Sage leaves, 8 to 10 leaves

Directions:

1. Place the sage leaves into a quart canning jar and add water that has boiled until it covers the leaves. Pour the lid on the jar and let sit for 15 minutes.

2. You can use this tea as a gargle to help ease a sore or scratchy throat. Usually, the pain will ease up before you even finish your first cup. This can also be used for inflammations of the throat, tonsils, and mouth since the mucous membranes get soothed by the sage oil. A normal dose would be between three to four cups each day. Every time you take a sip, roll it around in your mouth before swallowing it.

Nutrition:

Calories 26

Sugar 2.0g

Protein 7.6g

Fat 3.2g

Autumn Tonic Tea

Preparation Time: 10 minutes

Cooking Time: 15 minutes

Servings: 2

Ingredients :

• Dried ginger root, 1 part

• Rosehip, 1 part

• Red clover, 2 parts

• Dandelion root and leaf, 2 parts

• Mullein leaf, 2 parts

• Lemon balm, 3 parts

• Nettle leaf, 4 parts

Directions:

1. Place all of these Ingredients above into a bowl. Stir everything together to mix well. Put into a glass jar with a lid and keep it in a dry place that stays cool.

2. When you want a cup of tea, place four cups of water into a pot. Let this come to a full rolling boil. Place the desired amount of tea blend into a tea strainer, ball, or bag and cover with boiling water. Let sit for 15 minutes. Strain out the herbs and drink it either cold or hot. If you like your tea sweet, add some agave syrup or date sugar.

Nutrition:

Calories 43

Sugar 3.8g

Protein 6.5g

Fat 3.9g

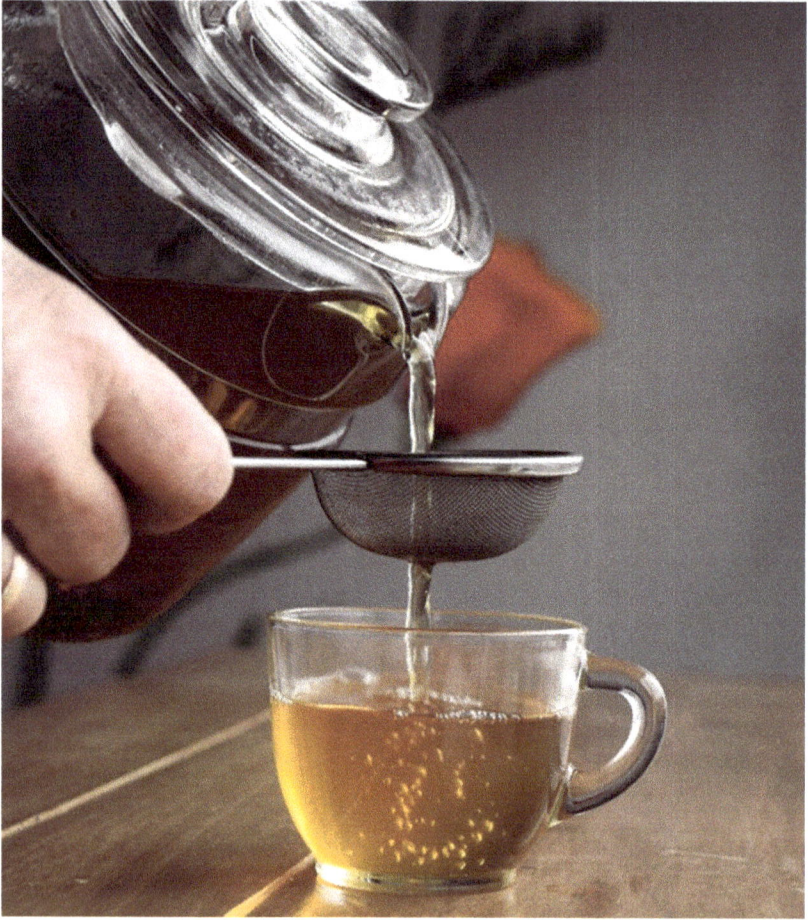

Adrenal And Stress Health

Preparation Time: 12 minutes

Cooking Time: 20 minutes

Servings: 2

Ingredients :

Bladder wrack, .5 c

Tulsi holy basil, 1 c

Shatavari root, 1 c

Ashwagandha root, 1 c

Directions:

1. Place these Ingredients into a bowl. Stir well to combine.

2. Place mixture in a glass jar with a lid and store in a dry place that stays cool.

3. When you want a cup of tea, place two tablespoons of the tea mixture into a medium pot. Pour in two cups of water. Let this come to a full rolling boil. Turn down heat. Let this simmer 20 minutes. Strain well. If you prefer your tea sweet, you can add some agave syrup or date sugar.

Nutrition:

Calories 43

Sugar 2.2g

Protein 4.1g

Fat 2.3g

Lavender Tea

Preparation Time: 5 minutes

Cooking Time: 15 minutes

Servings: 2

Ingredients :

• Agave syrup, to taste

• Dried lavender flowers, 2 tbsp.

• Fresh lemon balm, handful

• Water, 3 c

Directions:

1. Pour the water in a pot and allow to boil.

2. Pour over the lavender and lemon balm. Cover and let sit for five minutes.

3. Strain well. If you prefer your tea sweet, add some agave syrup.

Nutrition:

Calories 59

Sugar 6.8g

Protein 3.3g

Fat 1.6g

Choco-Nut Milkshake

Preparation Time: 10 minutes
Cooking Time: 0 minute
Servings: 2

Ingredients

• 2 cups unsweetened coconut, almond

• 1 banana, sliced and frozen

• ¼ cup unsweetened coconut flakes

• 1 cup ice cubes

• ¼ cup macadamia nuts, chopped

• 3 tablespoons sugar-free sweetener

• 2 tablespoons raw unsweetened cocoa powder

• Whipped coconut cream

Directions:

1. Place all Ingredients into a blender and blend on high until smooth and creamy.

2. Divide evenly between 4 "mocktail" glasses and top with whipped coconut cream, if desired.

3. Add a cocktail umbrella and toasted coconut for added flair.

4. Enjoy your delicious Choco-nut smoothie!

Nutrition:

12g Carbohydrates

3g Protein

199 Calories

Pineapple & Strawberry Smoothie

Preparation Time: 7 minutes

Cooking Time: 0 minute

Servings: 2

Ingredients :

• 1 cup strawberries

• 1 cup pineapple, chopped

• ¾ cup almond milk

• 1 tablespoon almond butter

Directions:

1. Add all Ingredients to a blender.

2. Blend until smooth.

3. Add more almond milk until it reaches your desired consistency.

4. Chill before serving.

Nutrition:

255 Calories

39g Carbohydrate

5.6g Protein

Cantaloupe Smoothie

Preparation Time: 11 minutes

Cooking Time: 0 minute

Servings: 2

Ingredients :

• ¾ cup carrot juice

• 4 cups cantaloupe, sliced into cubes

• Pinch of salt

• Frozen melon balls

• Fresh basil

Directions:

1. Add the carrot juice and cantaloupe cubes to a blender. Sprinkle with salt.

2. Process until smooth.

3. Transfer to a bowl.

4. Chill in the refrigerator for at least 30 minutes.

5. Top with the frozen melon balls and basil before serving.

Nutrition:

135 Calories

31g Carbohydrate

3.4g Protein

Berry Smoothie with Mint

Preparation Time: 7 minutes

Cooking Time: 0 minute

Servings: 2

Ingredients :

• ¼ cup orange juice

• ½ cup blueberries

• ½ cup blackberries

• 1 cup reduced-fat plain kefir

• 1 tablespoon honey

• 2 tablespoons fresh mint leaves

Directions:

1. Add all the Ingredients to a blender.

2. Blend until smooth.

Nutrition:

137 Calories

27g Carbohydrate

6g Protein

Green Smoothie

Preparation Time: 12 minutes

Cooking Time: 0 minute

Servings: 2

Ingredients :

• 1 cup vanilla almond milk (unsweetened)

• ¼ ripe avocado, chopped

• 1 cup kale, chopped

• 1 banana

• 2 teaspoons honey

• 1 tablespoon chia seeds

• 1 cup ice cubes

Directions:

1. Combine all the Ingredients in a blender.

2. Process until creamy.

Nutrition:

343 Calories

14.7g Carbohydrate

5.9g Protein

Banana, Cauliflower & Berry Smoothie

Preparation Time: 9 minutes

Cooking Time: 0 minute

Servings: 2

Ingredients :

• 2 cups almond milk (unsweetened)

• 1 cup banana, sliced

• ½ cup blueberries

• ½ cup blackberries

• 1 cup cauliflower rice

• 2 teaspoons maple syrup

Directions:

1. Pour almond milk into a blender.

2. Stir in the rest of the Ingredients.

3. Process until smooth.

4. Chill before serving.

Nutrition:

149 Calories

29g Carbohydrate

3g Protein

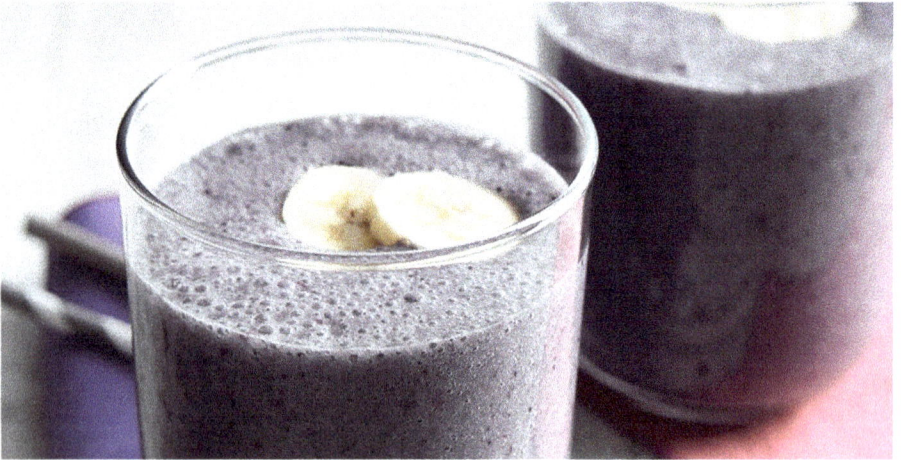

Berry & Spinach Smoothie

Preparation Time: 11 minutes

Cooking Time: 0 minute

Servings: 2

Ingredients :

• 2 cups strawberries

• 1 cup raspberries

• 1 cup blueberries

• 1 cup fresh baby spinach leaves

• 1 cup pomegranate juice

• 3 tablespoons milk powder (unsweetened)

Directions:

1. Mix all the Ingredients in a blender.

2. Blend until smooth.

3. Chill before serving.

Nutrition:

118 Calories

25.7g Carbohydrate

4.6g Protein

Peanut Butter Smoothie with Blueberries

Preparation Time: 12 minutes

Cooking Time: 0 minute

Servings: 2

Ingredients :

• 2 tablespoons creamy peanut butter

• 1 cup vanilla almond milk (unsweetened)

• 6 oz. soft silken tofu

• ½ cup grape juice

• 1 cup blueberries

• Crushed ice

Directions:

1. Mix all the Ingredients in a blender.

2. Process until smooth.

Nutrition:

247 Calories

30g Carbohydrate

10.7g Protein

Peach & Apricot Smoothie

Preparation Time: 11 minutes

Cooking Time: 0 minute

Servings: 2

Ingredients :

• 1 cup almond milk (unsweetened)

• 1 teaspoon honey

• ½ cup apricots, sliced

• ½ cup peaches, sliced

• ½ cup carrot, chopped

• 1 teaspoon vanilla extract

Directions:

1. Mix milk and honey.

2. Pour into a blender.

3. Add the apricots, peaches and carrots.

4. Stir in the vanilla.

5. Blend until smooth.

Nutrition:

153 Calories

30g Carbohydrate

32.6g Protein

Tropical Smoothie

Preparation Time: 8 minutes

Cooking Time: 0 minute

Servings: 2

Ingredients :

• 1 banana, sliced

• 1 cup mango, sliced

• 1 cup pineapple, sliced

• 1 cup peaches, sliced

• 6 oz. nonfat coconut yogurt

• Pineapple wedges

Directions:

1. Freeze the fruit slices for 30 minutes.

2. Transfer to a blender.

3. Stir in the rest of the Ingredients except pineapple wedges.

4. Process until smooth.

5. Garnish with pineapple wedges.

Nutrition:

102 Calories

22.6g Carbohydrate

2.5g Protein

Banana & Strawberry Smoothie

Preparation Time: 7 minutes

Cooking Time: 0 minute

Servings: 2

Ingredients :

• 1 banana, sliced

• 4 cups fresh strawberries, sliced

• 1 cup ice cubes

• 6 oz. yogurt

• 1 kiwi fruit, sliced

Directions:

1. Add banana, strawberries, ice cubes and yogurt in a blender.

2. Blend until smooth.

3. Garnish with kiwi fruit slices and serve.

Nutrition:

54 Calories

11.8g Carbohydrate

1.7g Protein

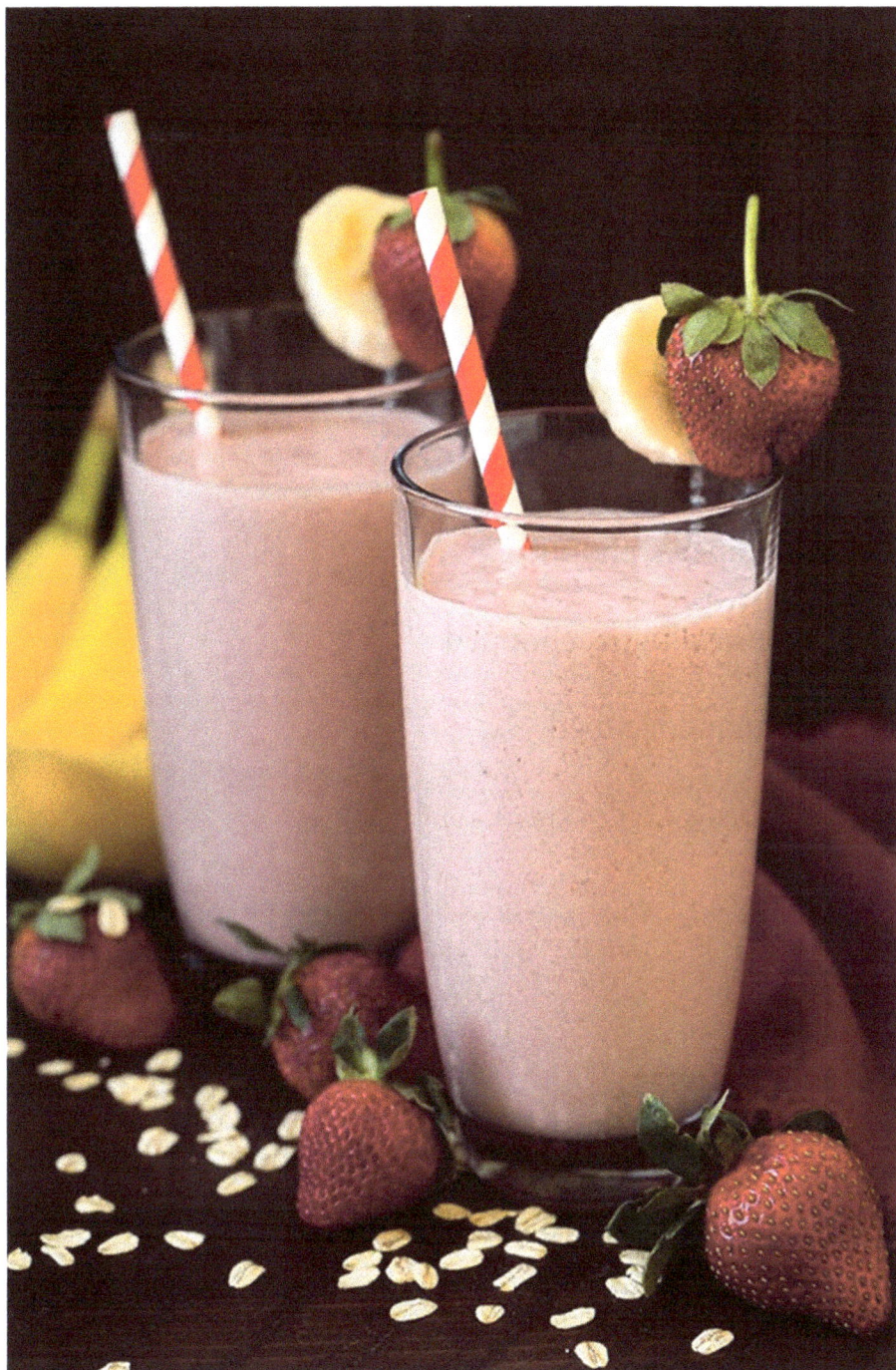

Cantaloupe & Papaya Smoothie

Preparation Time: 9 minutes
Cooking Time: 0 minute
Servings: 2

Ingredients :

• ¾ cup low-fat milk

• ½ cup papaya, chopped

• ½ cup cantaloupe, chopped

• ½ cup mango, cubed

• 4 ice cubes

• Lime zest

Directions:

1. Pour milk into a blender.

2. Add the chopped fruits and ice cubes.

3. Blend until smooth.

4. Garnish with lime zest and serve.

Nutrition:

207 Calories

18. 4g Carbohydrate

7. 7g Protein

Green Fruit Juice

Preparation Time: 10 minutes

Cooking Time: 0 minutes

Servings: 2

Ingredients :

• 3 large kiwis, peeled and chopped

• 3 large green apples, cored and sliced

• 2 cups seedless green grapes

• 2 teaspoons fresh lime juice

Directions:

Add all Ingredients into a juicer and extract the juice according to the manufacturer's method.

Pour into 2 glasses and serve immediately.

Nutrition:

Calories 304

Total Fat 2.2 g

Saturated Fat 0 g

Protein 6.2 g

Kale Chickpea Mash

Kale and chickpea produce a healthy and yummy lunch dish that has a wide range of ghealth benefits. It's perfect for people on the alkaline diet.

Preparation Time: 15 minutes
Cooking Time: 12 minutes
Servings: 1

Ingredients :

- 1 shallot

- 3 tbsp garlic

- A bunch of kale

- 1/2 cup boiled chickpea

- 2 tbsp coconut oil

- Sea salt

Directions:

1. Add some garlic in olive oil

2. Chop shallot and fry it with oil in a nonstick skillet.

3. Cook until the shallot turns golden brown.

4. Add kale and garlic in the skillet and stir well.

5. Add chickpeas and cook for 6 minutes. Add the rest of the Ingredients and give a good stir.

6. Serve and enjoy

Nutrition:

Calories: 149

Total fat: 8 grams

Saturated fat: 1 grams

Net carbohydrates: 13 grams

Protein: 4 grams

Sugars 6g

Fiber 3g

Sodium 226mg

Potassium 205mg

Quinoa And Apple

The combination of quinoa and apple yields a delicious and filling lunch dish that can be carried to work in your lunch box.

Preparation Time: 15 minutes
Cooking Time: 12 minutes
Servings: 1

Ingredients :

• 1/2 cup quinoa

• 1 apple

• 1/2 lemon

• Cinnamon to taste

Directions:

1. Cook quinoa according to the packet Directions.

2. Grate the apple and add to the cooked quinoa. Cook for 30 seconds.

3. Serve in a bowl then sprinkle lime and cinnamon. Enjoy.

Nutrition:

Calories 229

Total fat: 3.2 grams

Net carbs: 32.3 grams

Protein: 6.1 grams

Sugars: 4.2 grams

Fiber: 3.3 grams

Sodium: 35.5 milligrams

Potassium: 211. 8 milligrams

Warm Avo And Quinoa Salad

This is an amazing alkaline quinoa dish that will blow your mind away. It's an easy dish that will be ready in less than 20 minutes.

Preparation Time: 5 minutes
Cooking Time: 12 minutes
Servings: 4

Ingredients :

• 4 ripe avocados, quartered

• 1 cup quinoa

• 0.9 lb. Chickpeas, drained

• 1 oz flat leaf parsley

Directions:

1. Add quinoa in a pot with 2 cups of water.. Bring to boil then simmer for 12 minutes or until all the water has evaporated. The grains should be glassy and swollen.

2. Toss the quinoa with all other Ingredients and season with salt and pepper to taste.

3. Serve with olive oil and lemon wedges. Enjoy.

Nutrition:

Calories: 354

Total fat: 16 grams

Saturated fat: 2 grams

Net carbs: 31 grams

Protein: 15 grams

Sugars: 6 grams

Fiber: 15 grams

Sodium: 226 milligrams

Potassium: 205 milligrams

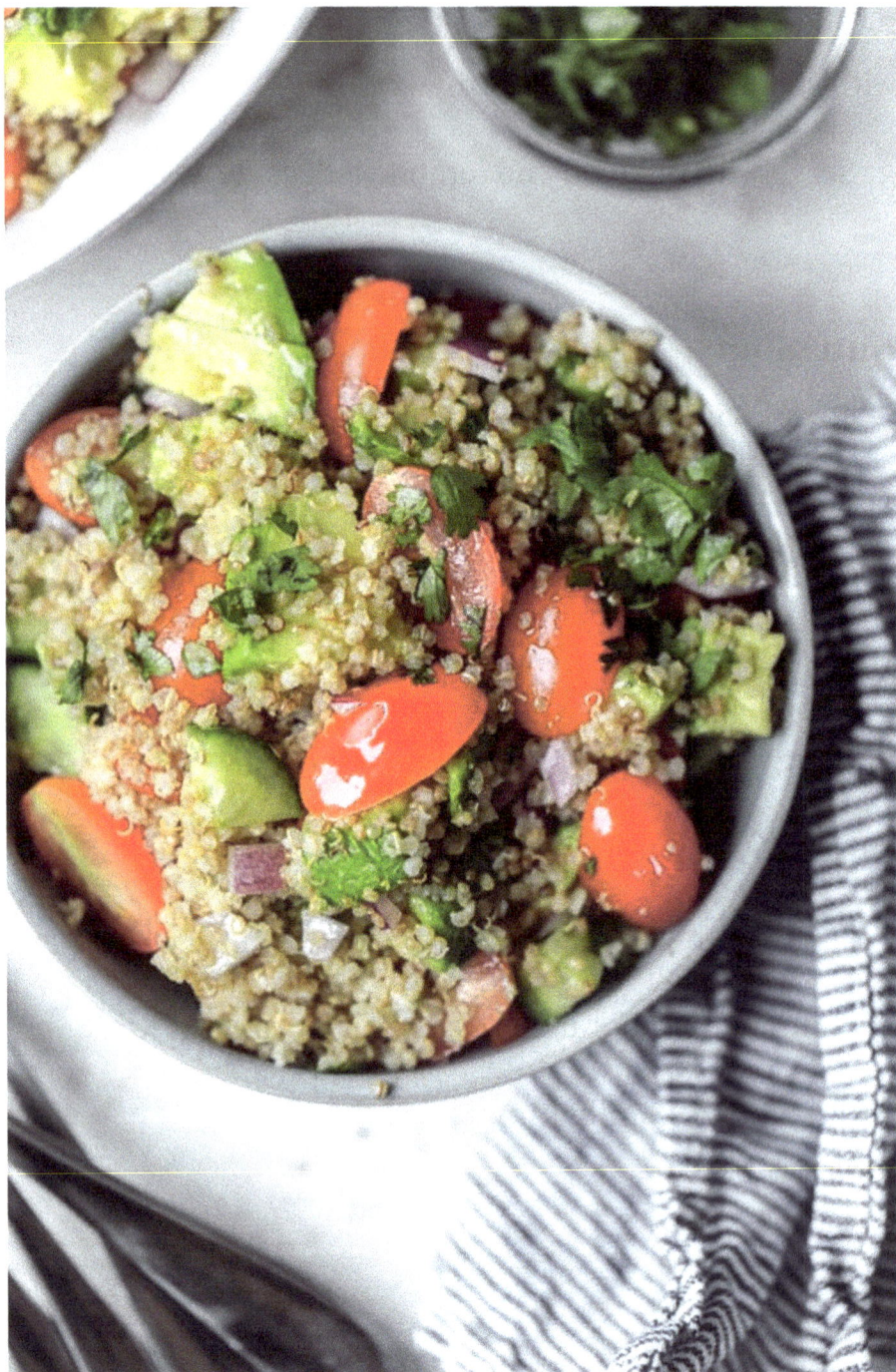

Spinach With Chickpeas And Lemon

If looking for an alkaline lunch to carry in your lunch box as part of a busy lifestyle, this flavorful easy recipe is the one for you.

Preparation Time: 5 minute
Cooking Time: 10 minutes
Servings: 2

Ingredients :

• 3 tbsp oil

• 1 onion, thinly slices

• 4 garlic cloves, minced

• 1 tbsp ginger, grated

• 1/2 container cherry tomatoes

• 1 lemon, freshly zested and juiced

• 1 tbsp red pepper flakes, crushed

• 1 can chickpeas

• Salt to taste

Directions:

1. Add oil in a skillet and cook onions until browned. Add garlic cloves, ginger, tomatoes, zest, and pepper flakes. Cook for 4 minutes.

2. Add chickpeas and cook for 3 more minutes. Add spinach and cook until they start to wilt.

3. Add lemon juice and season with salt to taste. Cook for 2 more minutes.

4. Serve and enjoy.

Nutrition:

Calories: 209

Total fat: 8.1 grams

Saturated fat: 1 grams

Total carbohydrates: 28.5 grams

Protein: 22.5 grams

Fiber: 6 grams

Sodium: 372 milligrams

Potassium: 286 milligrams

Raw Green Veggie Soup

A delightful and welcoming flavorsome soup that is completely energizing and uplifting especially during dr.sebi's diet.

Preparation Time: 5 minutes
Cooking Time: 5 minutes
Servings: 1

Ingredients :

• 1 avocado

• 1 zucchini, chopped

• 2 celery stalks, chopped

• 2 cups spinach

• 1/4 cup parsley, fresh

• 2 slices green pepper

• 1/8 onion, chopped

• 1 garlic clove

• 1/4 cup almonds, soak overnight and rinse

- Salt to taste

- 1-1/2 cup water

- 1 lemon juice

- Diced watermelon radish for garnish

Directions:

1. Add all the Ingredients in a food processor except salt.

2. Pulse until smooth or until the desired consistency is desired.

3. Pour the soup in a sauce pan to warm a little bit before seasoning with salt and squeezing lemon.

4. Garnish with watermelon radish and enjoy.

Nutrition:

Calories 48.9

Total fat 0.4 grams

Saturated fat 0.1 grams

Total carbs 10.6 grams

Net carbs 6.7 grams

Protein 3.1 grams

Sugars 1.9 grams

Fiber 3.9 grams

Sodium 619 milligrams

Potassium 417 milligrams

Kale Caesar Salad

An easy and classic way to enjoy your kale during lunch time. The dish is filling and complements dr.sebi's diet.

Preparation Time: 5 minutes
Cooking Time: 12 minutes
Servings: 1

Ingredients :

• 1 bunch of curly kale, washed

• 1 cup sunflower seeds

• 1/3 cup almond nuts

• 1/8 tbsp chipotle powder

• 2 garlic cloves

• 1-1/4 water

• 1-1/2 tbsp agave syrup

• 1/2 tbsp sea salt

Directions:

1. Wash and pat dry the curly kale and remove the center membrane .tear the kale leaves into small sizes.

2. Add all other Ingredients in a blender and blend until smooth and creamy.

3. Pour half of the mixture over the kale and toss until well coated.

4. Pour the remaining mixture and mix until the kales are well coated on the curls and folds.

5. Let rest for 10 minutes then serve on plates. Sprinkle sunflower seeds and enjoy.

Nutrition:

Calories: 157

Total fat: 6 grams

Saturated fat: 2 grams

Total carbohydrates: 18 grams

Protein: 9 grams

Sugars: 1 grams

Fiber: 2 grams

Sodium: 356 milligrams

Red And White Salad

The macadamia nuts and avocado oil add a beautiful buttery flavor to this salad. You can also use your favorite nuts and oil.

Preparation Time: 5 minutes
Cooking Time: 10 minutes
Servings: 2

Ingredients :

• 3 radishes

• 1 fennel bulb, greens removed

• 1/2 jicama, peeled and halved

• 2 celery stalks

• Juice from 1 lime

• 1/4 cup avocado oil

• Salt to taste

• Macadamia nuts

Directions:

1. Slice radish, fennel, jicama and celery using a mandolin slicer on the thinnest setting.

2. Toss them in a mixing bowl with lime and oil. Season with salt then top with nuts.

Enjoy.

Nutrition:

Calories: 197

Total fat: 9 grams

Saturated fat: 4 grams

Total carbs: 20 grams

Protein: 7 grams

Sugars: 1 gram

Fiber: 2 grams

Sodium: 366 milligrams

Arugula, Strawberry, & Orange Salad

Preparation Time: 15 minutes

Cooking Time: 15 minutes

Servings: 4

Ingredients :

• Salad

• 6 cups fresh baby arugula

• 1½ cups fresh strawberries, hulled and sliced

• 2 oranges, peeled and segmented

Dressing

• 2 tablespoons fresh lemon juice

• 1 tablespoon raw honey

• 2 teaspoons extra-virgin olive oil

• 1 teaspoon Dijon mustard

• Salt and ground black pepper, to taste

Directions:

• For salad: in a salad bowl, place all Ingredients and mix.

• For dressing: place all Ingredients in another bowl and beat until well combined.

• Place dressing on top of salad and toss to coat well.

• Serve immediately.

Nutrition:

Calories 107

Total Fat 2.9 g

Saturated Fat 0.4 g

Cholesterol 0 mg

Protein 2.1 g

Almond Milk

This is an awesome alternative to cow milk that is healthy, cheap and very easy to make. Serve the milk with your favorite alkaline side for a filling lunch.

Preparation Time: 5 minutes

Cooking Time: 10 minutes

Servings: 2

Ingredients :
- **1.** 7oz almonds, sliced

- 13**3.** 8 oz filtered water

- 1 tbsp sunflower granules

- 2 dates, stones removed

Directions:
1. Soak the almonds for a few minutes ahead of time.

2. Add all the Ingredients in a blender and blend for 2 minutes.

3. Pour the milk in a container through a straining cloth. Carry in your lunch box or store in a fridge for up to 3 days.

4. You can use almond pulp in cakes or almond mixes.

Nutrition:

Calories 90

Total fat: 2.5 grams

Total carbohydrates: 16 grams

Protein: 1 grams

Sugars: 4 grams

Sodium: 140 milligrams

Potassium: 140 milligrams

Creamy Kale Salad With Avocado And Tomato

This alkaline bowl is healthy, delicious, and filling. It's also very easy to assemble and can be carried to work in your lunchbox.

Preparation Time: 5 minutes

Cooking Time: 10 minutes

Servings: 2

Ingredients :

• 2 handful of kale

• 2 cherry tomatoes

• 1 ripe avocado

• Juice from 1 lime

• 1 garlic clove, crushed

• 1 tbsp agave

• 1/2 tbsp paprika

• 1/2 tbsp black pepper

Directions:

1. Wash kale and tomatoes and roughly chop them. Place them in a mixing bowl.

2. Peel the avocado and add it to the mixing bowl.

3. Add lemon juice and the rest of the Ingredients to the bowl and mix them thoroughly.

4. Serve and enjoy.

Nutrition:

Calories: 179.2

Total fat: 14.1 grams

Saturated fat: 1.9 grams

Total carbohydrates: 13.5 grams

Protein: 3.7 grams

Sugars: 6 grams

Fiber: 6.1 grams

Sodium: 77 milligrams

Potassium: 624 milligrams

Creamy Broccoli Soup

This is a thick and flavorful soup recipe. Its simple quick and the most delicious soup to serve for lunch.

Preparation Time: 5 minutes

Cooking Time: 10 minutes

Servings: 5

Ingredients :

• 2 cups vegetable stock

• 4 cups broccoli, chopped

• 1 red pepper, chopped

• 1 avocado

• 2 onions, chopped

• 2 celery stalks, sliced

• Ginger to taste

• 1 tbsp salt

Directions:

1. Warm vegetable stock in a small pot. Add broccoli and season with salt to taste. Simmer for 5 minutes.

2. Add the broccoli in a blender with pepper, avocado, onions, and celery stalks. Add some water for thinning then blend until smooth.

3. Serve when warm with ginger to your liking. Garnish with a lemon slice. Enjoy.

Nutrition:

Calories: 270

Total fat: 18 grams

Saturated fat: 11 grams

Total carbohydrates: 17 grams

Protein: 12 grams

Sugars: 5 grams

Fiber: 3.5 grams

Sodium: 470 milligrams

Beef & Kale Salad

Preparation Time: 15 minutes

Cooking Time: 8 minutes

Servings: 2

Ingredients :

Steak

• 2 teaspoons olive oil

• 2 (4-ounce) strip steaks

• Salt and ground black pepper, to taste

Salad

• ¼ cup carrot, peeled and shredded

• ¼ cup cucumber, peeled, seeded, and sliced

• ¼ cup radish, sliced

• ¼ cup cherry tomatoes, halved

• 3 cups fresh kale, tough ribs removed and chopped

Dressing

- 1 tablespoon extra-virgin olive oil

- 1 tablespoon fresh lemon juice

- Salt and ground black pepper, to taste

Directions:

1. For steak: in a large heavy-bottomed wok, heat the oil over high heat and cook the steaks with salt and black pepper for about 3–4 minutes per side.

2. Transfer the steaks onto a cutting board for about 5 minutes before slicing.

3. For salad: place all Ingredients in a salad bowl and mix.

4. For dressing: place all Ingredients in another bowl and beat until well combined.

5. Cut the steaks into desired sized slices against the grain.

6. Place the salad onto each serving plate.

7. Top each plate with steak slices.

8. Drizzle with dressing and serve.

Nutrition:

Calories 262

Total Fat 12 g

Saturated Fat 1.6 g

Protein 25.2 g

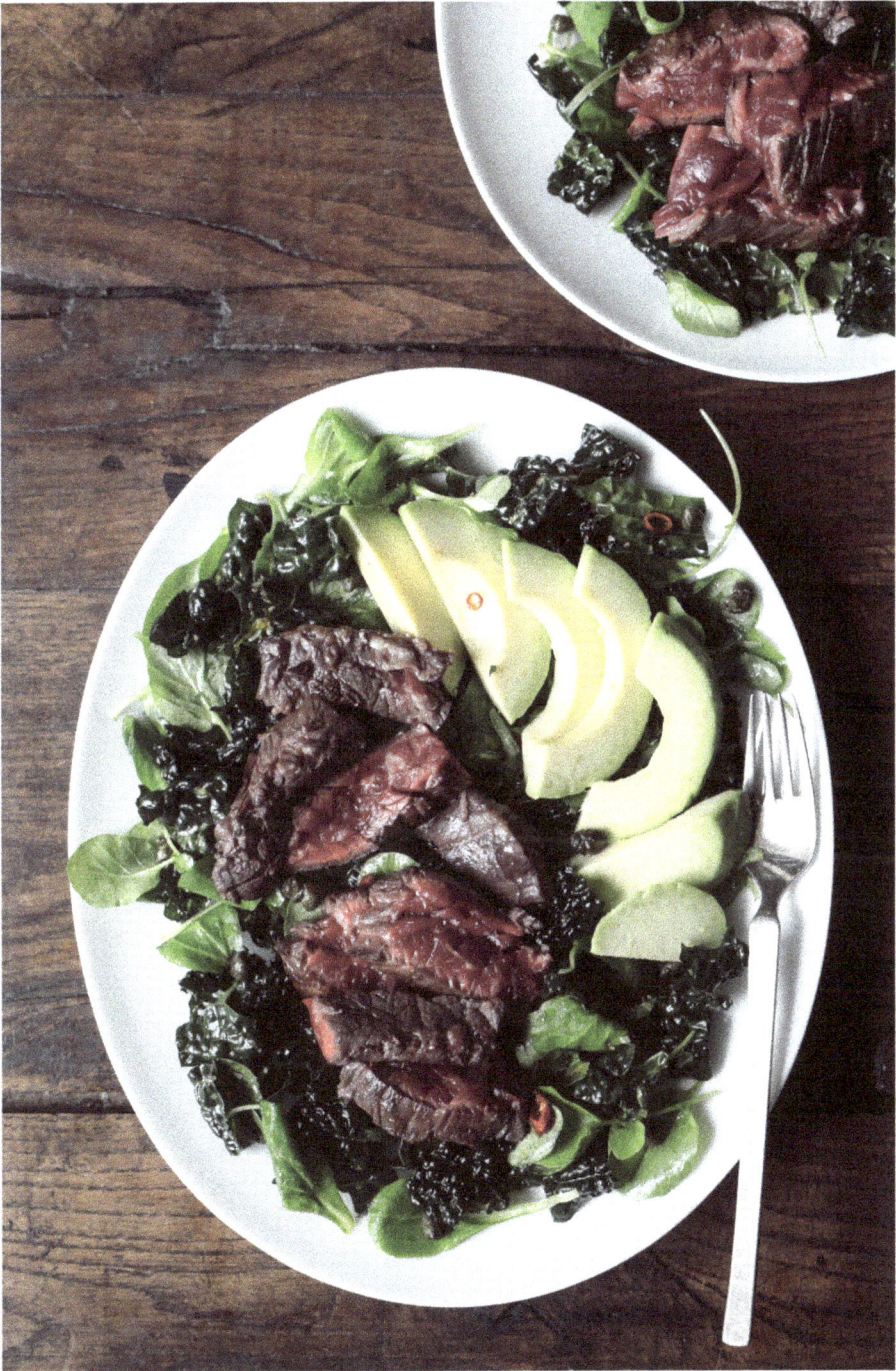

Capress Stuffed Avocado

The sweet juicy cherry tomatoes are tossed in basil pesto together with boccoccini balls then stuffed in avocado halves for a delightful light lunch.

Preparation Time: 5 minutes
Cooking Time: 10 minutes
Servings: 4

Ingredients :

• 1/2 cup cherry tomatoes

• 4 oz baby bocconcini balls

• 2 tbsp basil pesto

• 1 tbsp minced garlic

• 1/4 oil

• Salt and pepper to taste

• 2 ripe avocados

• 2 tbsp balsamic glaze

• Basil for serving

Directions:

1. In a mixing bowl, add cherry tomatoes, bocconcini balls, basil pesto, garlic, salt and pepper to taste. Toss until well combined and all flavors have blended.

2. Half the avocados and arrange them on a platter.

3. Spoon the mixture in the avocado halves and drizzle with balsamic glaze.

4. Top with basil and serve. Enjoy.

Nutrition:

Calories: 341

Total fat: 29grams

Saturated fat: 7grams

Total carbohydrates: 15grams

Protein: 8 grams

Sugars: 4 grams

Fiber: 6 grams

Sodium: 220 milligrams

Potassium: 550 milligrams

Alkaline Mushroom Chickpea Burgers Recipe

Preparation Time: 20 minutes

Cooking Time: 30 minutes

Servings: 8

Ingredients :

• 2 portobello mushrooms

• 2 cups cooked chickpeas

• 2 tsp. Onion powder

• 2 tsp. Himalayan sea salt

• 2 tsp. Oregano

• 1/2 cup cilantro

• 1/4 cup garbanzo bean flour

• 1/2 tsp. Cayenne

• 1/2 cup green peppers

• 1/2 cup red and white onions

• Food processor or blender

- 1/4 measurement cup

Directions:

1. Chop the mushrooms into chunks and dice the vegetables.

2. Place all the Ingredients in a food processor and pulse for 3 seconds.

3. Check for consistency, if it's too wet, add more flour then scoop into a bowl.

4. Set your cooker to medium heat and sprinkle grapeseed oil into the skillet.

5. Scoop the blend into a cup and turn it over to your cooking surface.

6. Allow the blend to for 5 minutes on each side. Apply caution when flipping so that the blend can stay together.

7. Your alkaline mushroom/chickpea burgers is ready to be served.

Nutrition:

Calories: 225 calories

Carbohydrates: 22.5 grams

Fat: 14.2 grams

Protein: 11.4 grams

Alkaline Veggie Fajitas Recipe

Preparation Time: 10 minutes

Cooking Time: 20 minutes

Servings: 6-12

Ingredients :

Fixings:

• 1/2 cups cut green and red peppers

• 1/2 cups cut red and white onions

• 3 cups cut mushrooms

• 2 tsp. Ocean salt

• 2 tsp. Onion powder

• 2 tsp. Sweet basil

• 2 tsp. Oregano

• 1/2 tsp. Cayenne powder

• Juice from 1/2 of a lime

• Grapeseed oil

- Alkaline spelt tortillas

- Alkaline guacamole (discretionary)

- Alkaline mango salsa (discretionary)

- If you would prefer not to utilize mushrooms in this formula, you can essentially preclude them and cut each preparing down the middle

Directions:

1. Make your mushrooms, bell peppers and onions into long strips.

2. Set your cooker to medium heat then sprinkle a tablespoon of grapeseed oil on the skillet.

3. Sprinkle another tablespoon of grapeseed oil on a large skillet.

4. Mix your vegetables and seasoning, then, sauté for 5 minutes.

5. Serve them on spelt tortillas with the guacamole and salsa.

6. Your alkaline veggie fajitas is ready to be dished.

Nutrition:

Calories: 257

Fat: 2 grams

Saturated fat: 0.4 grams

Protein: **12.** 9 grams

Carbohydrate: 50.3 grams

Sugar: 8 grams

Alkaline Vegan Hot Dogs Recipe

Preparation Time: 20 minutes

Cooking Time: 40 minutes

Servings: 10

Ingredients :

• 1 cup garbanzo beans

• 1 cup spelt flour

• 1/2 cup aquafaba

• 1/3 cup green pepper, diced

• 1/3 cup onion, diced

• 1/4 cup shallots, diced

• 1 tbsp. Onion powder

• 2 tsp. Smoked sea salt

• 1 tsp. Coriander

• 1/2 tsp. Ginger

• 1/2 tsp. Dill

- 1/2 tsp. Fennel

- 1/2 tsp. Crushed red pepper (optional)

- Alkaline electric ketchup (optional)

- Grapeseed oil for sautéing

- Alkaline electric buns (optional)

****when trying to make hotdog buns, all you have to do is follow the recipe to roll the dough then bake on taco rack. In the absence of a rack, flatbread or tortillas can be used instead.****

Tools:

Hotdog mold

Food processor

Parchment paper

Taco rack (optional)

Directions:

1. Sprinkle grapeseed oil in your skillet, add vegetables and garbanzo beans then sauté for 5 minutes.

2. Place the remaining vegetables and other **Ingredients** in a food processor until it is well blended.

3. Scoop the mixture into your hand, then, make hotdog shapes with them and wrap with parchment paper afterwards.

4. The molded hotdogs should be steamed for 40 minutes.

5. Once the steaming process is done, unwrap the hotdogs.

6. Sprinkle grapeseed oil in a skillet and cook the hotdogs for 10 minutes on medium heat.

7. Your alkaline electric hotdogs is ready to be dished.

Nutrition:

Calories: 159.2

Carbohydrates: 6.3 grams

Fat: 3.3 grams

Protein: 25.5 grams

Alkaline Avocado Mayo Recipe

Preparation Time: 10 minutes

Cooking Time: 10 minutes

Servings: 1 cup

Ingredients :

• Juice from half of a lime

• 1 avocado

• 1/4 cup cilantro

• 1/2 tsp. Sea salt

• 1/2 tsp. Onion powder

• 2-4 tbsp. Olive oil

• Pinch of cayenne powder

• Blender or hand mixer

Directions:

1. Remove the pit of the avocado and scoop the insides into a blender.

2. Add the rest of the Ingredients and blend at a high speed.

3. For hand mixers, add all other Ingredients except the oil which should be added slowly until a desired consistency is reached.

4. Dish your alkaline avocado mayo!

Nutrition:

Calories: 45

Fat: 4.5 grams

Sodium: 100 milligrams

Carbohydrate: 0.5 gram

Alkaline Quinoa Milk Recipe

Preparation Time: 10 minutes

Cooking Time: 5 minutes

Servings: 4

Ingredients :

• 1 cup cooked white quinoa

• 3 cups spring water

• 6-8 dates

• 1 pinch sea salt (optional)

• 1 pinch cloves (optional)

• Blender

• Milk bag or cheese cloth

Directions:

1. Make a perfect blend of these Ingredients in a blender.

2. Sieve with milk bag or cheesecloth.

3. Enjoy your well-deserved alkaline quinoa milk recipe.

Nutrition:

Calories: 111

Sugar: 3.2 grams

Sodium: 5 milligrams

Fat: 1.6 grams

Saturated fat: 0.2 grams

Carbohydrates: 20.7 grams

Fiber: 2.3 grams

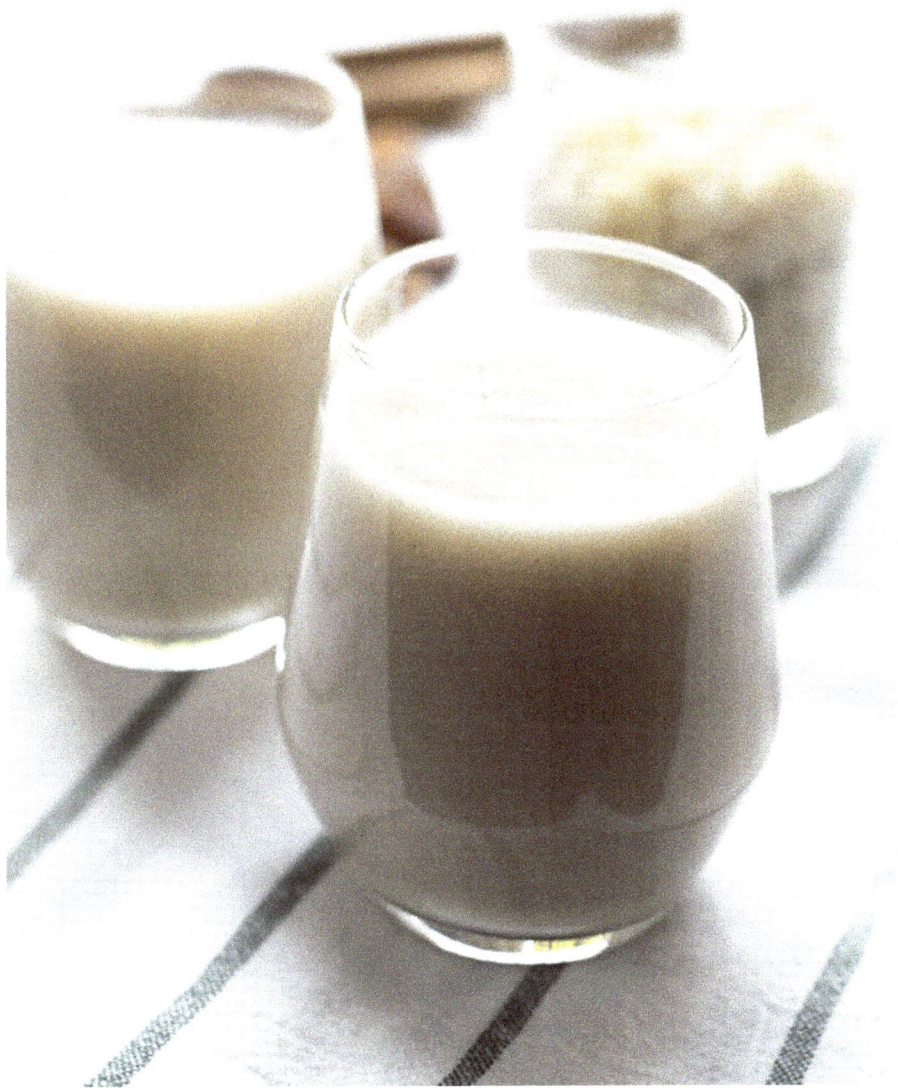

Spicy Kale Recipe

Preparation Time: 10 minutes

Cooking Time: 15 minutes

Servings: 4

Ingredients :

• 1 bunch of kale

• 1/4 cup onion, diced

• 1/4 cup red pepper, diced

• 1 tsp. Crushed red pepper

• 1/4 tsp. Sea salt

• Alkaline "garlic" oil or grape seed oil

• Salad spinner (optional)

• Note: if you happen to not have a salad spinner, you can as well air dry the kale.

Directions:

1. Rinse the kale, fold its leaves into halves and cut off the stem.

2. Chop kale into bits and remove the water using a salad spinner.

3. Set your cooker to high and add 2 tablespoon of oil.

4. Sauté salt, pepper and onions for 3 minutes.

5. Reduce the heat to low, add the chopped kale and cover for 5 minutes.

6. Crushed pepper should be introduced to the mix, stir and cover for another 3 minutes.

7. Dish your alkaline spicy kale!

Nutrition:

Calories: 85.2

Fat: 1.2 grams

Sodium: 61.2 milligrams

Carbohydrates: 18 grams

Fiber: 5.9 grams

Protein: 5.3 grams

Alkaline Buns Recipe

Preparation Time: 20 minutes

Cooking Time: 40 minutes

Servings: 6

Ingredients :

• 2 1/4 cups - 2 1/2 cups spelt flour

• 1/2 cup hemp milk or walnut milk

• 1/4 cup aquafaba

• 1/4 cup sparkling spring water

• 1 tbsp. Agave

• 1 tbsp. Onion powder

• 1 1/2 tsp. Sea salt

• 1 tsp. Basil or oregano

• 2 tsp. Grapeseed oil

• 1 tsp. Sea moss gel (optional)

• Sesame seeds (optional)

- Mixer with dough hook*

- Baking sheet

- Plastic wrap

- Parchment paper

- Note: if you do not have a mixer, you can knead by hand.

Directions:

1. Add all the dry Ingredients into a mixing bowl and blend perfectly.

2. Add the remaining Ingredients and blend on low speed for a minute. Then, knead dough at medium speed for 5 minutes.

3. Sprinkle grapeseed oil on a baking sheet already laced with parchment paper.

4. Separate dough into parts, roll with hand to make shapes then place on baking sheet.

5. Brush the top with oil then add sesame seeds.

6. Use a plastic wrap to cover the buns and allow it to sit for 30 minutes.

7. Set your oven to 350°f and bake for 30 minutes.

8. Allow the buns to cook and carefully cut them in half to enjoy your alkaline electric buns!

Nutrition:

Carbohydrates: 47 grams

Fat: 7 grams

Protein: 9 grams

Alkaline Strawberry Jam Recipe

Preparation Time: 10 minutes

Cooking Time: 20 minutes

Servings: 16 oz

Ingredients :

• 4 cups sliced strawberries

• **Servings:** cups of raw agave

• 3 tablespoons of key lime juice

• 1/2 cup irish moss gel

Directions:

1. Slice enough strawberries to fill up 4 cups.

2. Mash or blend to your desired texture.

3. Agave, lime juice and strawberries should be added to the sauce pan on high heat.

4. Cook for 10 minutes then add irish moss gel.

5. Cook for 5 more minutes to make certain that the gel has been thoroughly dissolved.

6. Remove from heat and allow the sauce to cool down before refrigerating.

7. Dish your alkaline electric strawberry jam!

Nutrition:

Calories: 56

Carbohydrate: 13 grams

Alkaline Date Syrup Recipe

Preparation Time: 10 minutes

Cooking Time: 15 minutes

Servings: 16-24 oz

Ingredients :

• 1 cup dates, preferably pitted

• 1 cup of spring water

• This sweetener can be easily dissolved in water unlike date sugar.

Directions:

1. Boil spring water then remove from heat when boiled.

2. Place dates in the boiled water for at least 5 minutes.

3. Pour the dates and some water into a blender then blend for until it's smooth.

4. If the texture is too thick, add more water and blend again.

5. Keep it a refrigerator and dish with alkaline date syrup!

Nutrition:

Calories: 270

Potassium: 848 milligrams

Sodium: 5 milligrams

Carbohydrates: 67 grams

Fiber: 3 grams

Sugar: 61 grams

Protein: 1 grams

Chickpea Mashed Potatoes

Preparation Time: 5 minutes

Cooking Time: 30 minutes

Servings: 4

Ingredients :

• 2 cups chickpeas, cooked

• ¼ cup green onions, diced

• 2 teaspoons sea salt

• 2 teaspoons onion powder

• 1 cup walnut milk; homemade, unsweetened

Directions:

1. Plug in a food processor, add chickpeas to it, pour in the milk, and then add salt and onion powder.

2. Cover the blending jar with its lid and then pulse for 1 to 2 minutes until smooth; blend in water if the mixture is too thick.

3. Take a medium saucepan, place it over medium heat, and then add blended chickpea mixture in it.

4. Stir green onions into the chickpeas mixture and then cook the mixture for 30 minutes, stirring constantly.

5. Serve straight away.

Nutrition:

Calories: 145.8

Carbohydrates: 19.1 grams

Fat: 7.3 grams

Protein: 3.3 grams

Mushroom And Onion Gravy

Preparation Time: 5 minutes

Cooking Time: 18 minutes

Servings: 4

Ingredients :

- 1 cup sliced onions, chopped

- 1 cup mushrooms, sliced

- 2 teaspoons onion powder

- 2 teaspoons sea salt

- 1 teaspoon dried thyme

- 6 tablespoons chickpea flour

- ½ teaspoon cayenne pepper

- 1 teaspoon dried oregano

- 4 tablespoons grapeseed oil

- 4 cups spring water

Directions:

1. Take a medium pot, place it over medium-high heat, add oil and when hot, add onions and mushrooms, and then cook for 1 minute.

2. Season the vegetables with onion powder, salt, thyme, and oregano. Stir until mixed, and cook for 5 minutes.

3. Pour in water, stir in cayenne pepper, stir well, and then bring the mixture to a boil.

4. Slowly stir in chickpea flour, and bring the mixture to a boil again.

5. Remove pan from heat and then serve gravy with a favorite dish.

Nutrition:

Calories: 120

Carbohydrates: 8.4 grams

Fat: 7.6 grams

Protein: 2.2 grams

Vegetable Chili

Preparation Time: 5 minutes
Cooking Time: 30 minutes
Servings: 6

Ingredients :

• 2 cups black beans, cooked

• 1 medium red bell pepper; deseeded, chopped

• 1 poblano chili; deseeded, chopped

• 2 jalapeño chilies; deseeded, chopped

• 4 tablespoons cilantro, chopped

• 1 large white onion; peeled, chopped

• 1 ½ tablespoon minced garlic

• 1 ½ teaspoon sea salt

• 1 ½ teaspoon cumin powder

• 1 ½ teaspoon red chili powder

• 3 teaspoons lime juice

- 2 tablespoons grapeseed oil

- 2 ½ cups vegetable stock

Directions:

1. Take a large pot, place it over medium-high heat, add oil and when hot, add onion and cook for 4−5 minutes until translucent.

2. Add bell pepper, jalapeno pepper, poblano chili, and garlic and then cook for 3−4 minutes until veggies turn tender.

3. Season the vegetables with salt, stir in cumin powder and red chili powder, then add chickpeas and pour in vegetable stock.

4. Bring the mixture to a boil, then switch heat to medium-low and simmer the chili for 15−20 minutes until thickened slightly.

5. Then remove the pot from heat, ladle chili stew among six bowls, drizzle with lime juice, garnish with cilantro, and serve.

Nutrition:

Calories: 224.2

Carbs: 42.6 grams

Fat: 1.2 grams

Protein: 12.5 grams.

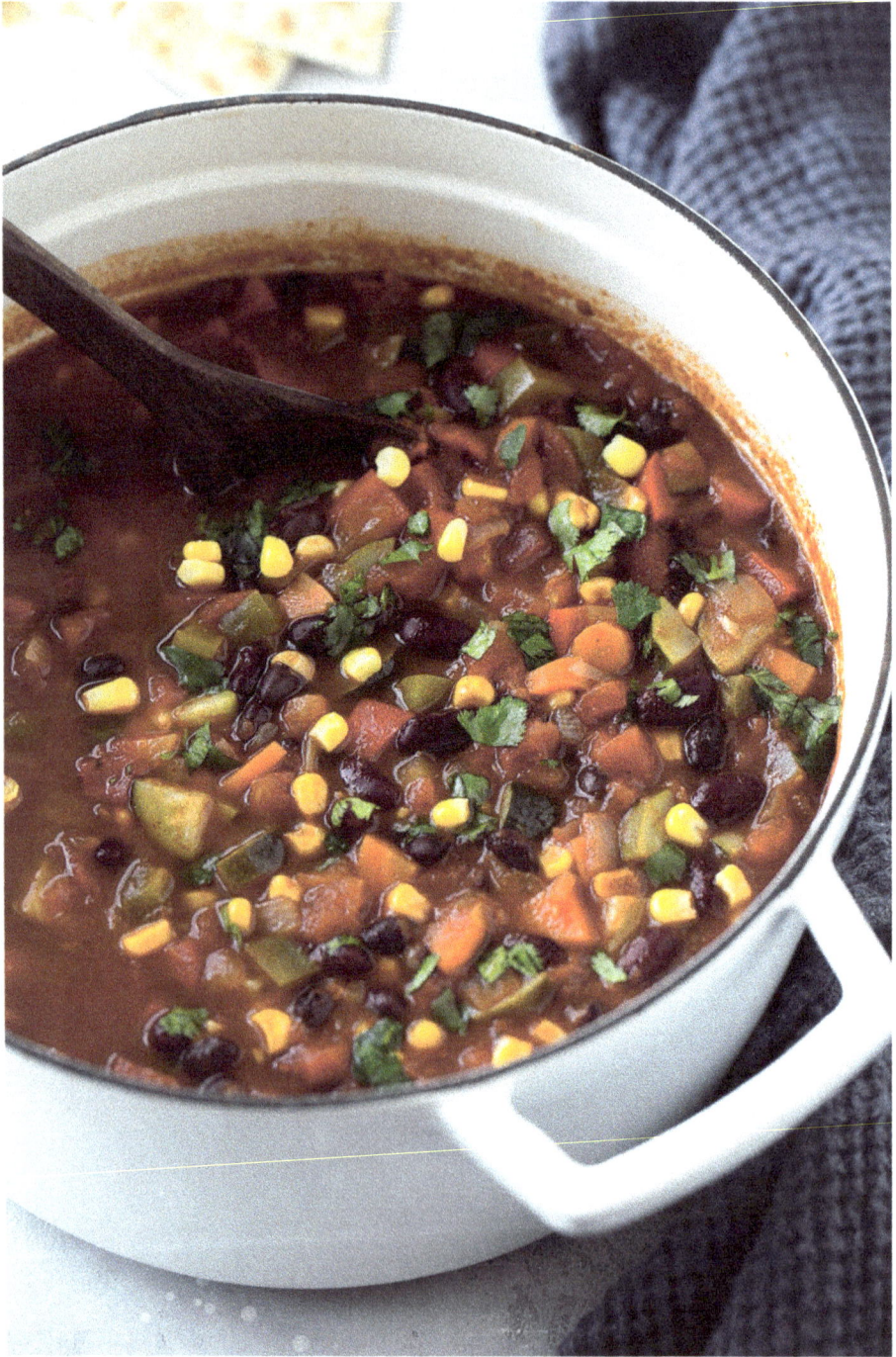

www.ingramcontent.com/pod-product-compliance
Lightning Source LLC
Chambersburg PA
CBHW050753030426
42336CB00012B/1800